LESS
PAIN
MORE
GAINS

SHORT THEORY – EFFECTIVE APPLICATION

FOR BUSY PEOPLE LOOKING TO FEEL HEALTHIER, HAPPIER, IMPROVE FITNESS LEVELS AND ACHIEVE FAT LOSS RESULTS FOR LIFE

EMMIR MORAN GOMEZ

Contents

To my grandmother Zoila, my mother Angelica, my wife Nina and her family, my family, the Mindset family, my friends and all the people who believe in me.

To you who will read this book.

Thank you.

About The Mindset

History

Back in Peru in 2014, The Mindset was created after overcoming, eating disorders and body image confident by a desire to contribute, serve and give back to the community. Emmir Moran Gomez took the decision to be the founder of this fitness movement.

Mission

The Mindset has a mission in this world to help you unlock your best, enjoy life and live longer. We are ready to take you to the next level physically, mentally and spiritually.

Who is The Mindset for?

The Mindset family is for everyone. We don't look for perfection, we look for a desire to unlock your best version of you. We will add experience, motivation, love, care and support.

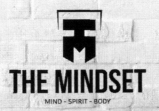

LOVE, SERVE AND IMPROVE EVERY DAY

THE MINDSET

MIND - SPIRIT - BODY

Introduction

It is the second lockdown of the coronavirus pandemic of 2020. Feeling frustrated and helpless, having a white board in front of me, I start writing down the things that made my athletes hire me and the common questions people ask me. I asked myself *how can I put all my knowledge and tools in one place*?

All the people I've worked with want to lose fat and feel better, but they don't have time or motivation. There is also so much information out there that it is confusing to understand what is right.

For that reason, I decided to write this book. This book will tell you the truth, the smart way to go and all the tools that you need to get there.

Your fitness journey has to be simple and easy, not complicated or hard to follow. This book is designed to be short and simple in theory and effective in application and guidelines.

Let me show you the new way to achieve your fitness goals and a lifetime of health and well-being.

Chapter One
Train Less – Achieve More

Why train less – achieve more?

The most effective exercises for stimulating muscle growth are multi-joint movements like squats, push ups, pull ups, steps up and so on. All the compound movements put a great deal of stress on the muscle which makes you burn more calories and also tone up in a faster way. Therefore, isolation movements like core or cardio are a waste of time if you are just focusing on them, as they are not targeting the full body. A better approach would be to add isolation movements, cardio exercise and compound movements in every training session.

To build an effective and quick training plan here is what you need to do:

Phase 1: Choose two compound movement exercises per big muscle group such as legs, back, shoulders and chest, then add one isolation movement exercise such as core and one cardiovascular exercise.

Example:

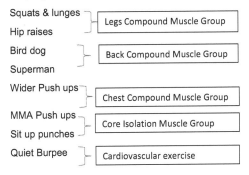

Squats & lunges ⎤
Hip raises   ⎦— Legs Compound Muscle Group

Bird dog   ⎤
Superman   ⎦— Back Compound Muscle Group

Wider Push ups ⎤
                ⎦— Chest Compound Muscle Group
MMA Push ups ⎤
Sit up punches ⎦— Core Isolation Muscle Group

Quiet Burpee ⎤— Cardiovascular exercise

Perform each exercise 3-4 times for 30-40 seconds each.

Phase 2: Add three exercises for warm up and three exercises for cool down.

Phase 3: You will perform this training three times a week. To make this training faster you could perform supersets, meaning you will do two exercises in a row, only taking a 30 second rest when you have completed both exercises.

Fat loss training plan example:

	Order	Exercises	Reps	Sets	Rest
Warm up	A	Neck & shoulder circles	3 times for 20 seconds each		
	B	Angel walls	3 times for 20 seconds each		
	C	Cow and cat	3 times for 20 seconds each		
Training Programme	Legs	Hip raises Squats & lunges	30-40 seconds 30-40 seconds	3-4	- 30 seconds
	Back	Bird dog Superman raises	30-40 seconds 30-40 seconds	3-4	- 30 seconds
	Chest	Wider push ups MMA push ups	30-40 seconds 30-40 seconds	3-4	- 30 seconds
	Core Cardio	Sit up punches Quiet burpee	30-40 seconds 30-40 seconds	3-4	- 30 seconds
Cool down	A	Kneeling back	30 seconds	3	-
	B	Knee to chest	30 seconds	3	-
	C	Auto hug	30 seconds	3	-

The duration of this training plan should be approximately 30 minutes for each session.

* go to page 59 to find pictures, examples and links to the videos for the exercises above.

Passive cardio is an easy way to burn more calories

Fat loss is not just about doing lots of cardio such as running or HIIT, it is about moving more and being more active than before. Let me ask you a question: which sport do you like the most? Maybe football, rugby, basketball or volleyball? Or how about trying a new sport that you haven't tried before? How about dancing? If you don't like any of these it's totally fine, you could also try walking. Yes, walking is the most secure and injury-free way to lose fat. You just need to make sure to achieve 10,000 steps per day between 2-4 times per week, which is around an hour walk on a normal to slow speed.

Action plan:
- Train 3 times a week for approximately 30 mins each session.
- Do any passive cardio of your choice for 2-4 times per week for an hour on your days off from training.

Wearing a smart fitness band helps me to track steps, target daily steps, track progress and have sedentary reminders. It's worth it!

My favourite brand is Xiaomi Mi Smart Band 4.

Chapter Two

No More Diets

How many times have you been starving yourself, steering away from bread and pasta and just eating salad every day?

Being hungry is a good sign that your body is working in an optimal level, however the key to eating more and having more fat loss results will be to focus on adding five important nutrients in every main meal you have.

Why?

Once you start to follow the training plan and become more active, you will need to fuel your body because you will be spending more energy. You need to imagine yourself like a car, if your car doesn't have petrol it will be really hard to get anywhere.

MIX AND MATCH FAT LOSS NUTRITION PLAN

PROTEIN (UNCOOKED)	CARBS (UNCOOKED)	VEGS/SALAD (UNLIMITED)	FAT	FRUIT
250G HIGH PROTEIN YOGURT 250G ALPRO SOYA YOGURT	30G GLUTEN FREE OATS	GARLIC, GINGER AND TUMERIC	15G OF NUT BUTTER	1 MEDIUM APPLE
2 MEDIUM WHOLE EGGS	2 MEDIUM SLICES OF WHOLEMEAL BREAD, 2 SOUR DOUGH, 2 RYE BREAD, 1 WHOLEMEAL WRAPS	SPINACH, KALE , GARDEN LEAFY GREENS	HALF A MEDIUM AVOCADO	250G PINEAPPLE
250ML SKIMMED MILK/ SOYA	60G QUINOA	GREEN BEANS	¼ TABLESPOON OF OLIVE OIL	2 KIWIS
150G CHICKEN BREAST	60G COUS COUS. BUCKWHEAT,BULGUR	BROCCOLI, CAULIFLOWER	15G OF NUTS	500G STRAWBERRIES
150G FILET COD/HAKE,TUNA,WHITE FISH	50G OF CHICKPEAS OR ANY LEGUME	BEETROOT	15G OF CHIA SEEDS	250G BERRIES (ANY)
200G KING PRAWNS, MIX SEA FOOD	50G WHOLEMEAL PASTA, SEMOLINA PASTA	ONION, PEPPERS	15G CHEDDAR CHEESE or ANY CHEESE	1 MEDIUM BANANA
150G FILLET SALMON	50G LENTILS (ANY TYPE)	ASPARAGUS,CUCUMBER	60G OF COTTAGE CHEESE	80G GRAPES
200G TURKEY BREAST /MINCE	50G OF RICE (ANY TYPE)	MIXED VEGETABLES, CARROTS, TOMTATOES		1 PLUM /PEACH / APRICOT
150G 5% FAT BEEF MINCE	1 MED SWEET POTATO / 150G NEW BABY POTATOES	ANY READY-MIXED SALAD (TESCO)		200G MELON /WATERMELON
1 SCOOP PROTEIN POWDER	200G ROOT VEGETABLES (DRIZZLE OF OLIVE OIL AND DRIZZLE OF HONEY)	MUSHROOMS		1 MEDIUM ORANGE

Yes, you can eat all of this!

Our bodies need every single nutrient on this chart. If we skip any of these our fat loss journey will be painful and not enjoyable at all. This may lead to us eating any food around us such as cookies and chips or even just coffee or plain salad sometimes. This food chart is designed to help you achieve your results in a faster way with the ideal quantities and I will show you how to you use it.

Mix and match nutritional plan guidelines

In the chart above you can see your nutritional meal plan which is designed to help you mix and match as you like in order to be ready for your food preparation. Here, you will have a variety of choices: protein, carbohydrates, fat, vegetables and fruit.

The purpose of this nutrition plan is to bring you the freedom to create a diet plan that works for you. In every meal choose one protein (uncooked), one carbohydrate (uncooked), unlimited vegetables or salad, one fat and finally one portion of fruit.

These need to be on every single plate.

If you're looking for fat loss, the best way to approach this mix and match nutrition plan is to have three main meals a day. You can have your meals at any time of day, however it's essential to cover all three meals.

Stick to the nutritional plan chart and accurately follow the information provided: sizes, grams, millilitres, drizzle, portions, type of bread/pasta etc.

Here some examples:

Meal One:

Alpro soya yogurt, 2 slices wholemeal bread, tomatoes, 1 medium banana, fresh sliced strawberries

Seasoning: Cinnamon

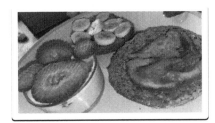

Meal Two:

60g middle eastern seasoned cous cous, half a medium avocado, broccoli, 1 medium Spanish chicken breast

Cous cous seasoning: garlic, paprika, nutmeg, cumin and pinch of salt

Chicken seasoning: bay leaf and paprika

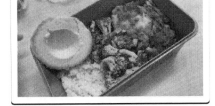

Meal Three:

1 fillet fresh seasoned salmon, 50g rice and mixed Mexican-seasoned vegetables

Salmon seasoning: lemon juice and parsley

Veg and rice seasoning: a pinch of black pepper and salt, a sprinkle of chilli powder, garlic

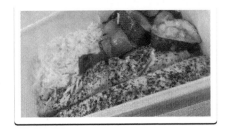

Note: Portion of fruit for meal two and three can be used as snacks during the day.

** *go to page 65 to find the nutritional guidelines video*

Chapter Three
Caffeine and Fat Loss

Many of us cannot live without caffeine and I totally understand; it is part of us, and I am not trying to take it away from you. Today I want to encourage you to have organic caffeine, natural caffeine, not a pill or product that will affect your nervous system and cognitive function making you dependent on it and not able to create energy for yourself.

Nowadays it is really common to have energy drinks, fat burners or any caffeine supplements and I get it. You need energy, yes or yes? But trust me, you will not need those supplements anymore as long as you are more active and have your five nutrients in every meal.

Why?

It is simply because when we move, we create energy and that energy we create will give us more energy for the rest of the day.

Let me give you an example. To generate electricity, or 'energy', you will need power stations. Turbines are turned using energy from sources such as heat, wind and moving water and that is how we convert motion (movement) into electrical energy. In the same way, food, water, breathing and sleep are the main energy sources you need to generate energy during the day. Just make sure to follow the nutritional guidelines in chapter two and *have at least 2 litres of water per day as a minimum intake.*

In the next two chapters I will give you tools to help with quality breathing (stress management) and sleep.

So, what do I mean when I talk about organic and natural caffeine? Let me give you some examples.

Natural caffeine alternatives:
A recommended amount of caffeine per day would be 4 cups before 6 p.m.

1. **Fresh ground coffee** (not granulated coffee): Use 2 tablespoons for every 180ml of water.
2. **Green tea**: Let the boiling water cool slightly before pouring onto the tea bag and allow to brew for 2 to 3 mins in 180ml of water.
3. **Chicory coffee**: Use 2 tablespoons of grounds for every 180ml of water.
4. **Matcha tea**: Sift 1-2 teaspoons of matcha powder into hot water and whisk together. A traditional bamboo tea whisk called a chasen works best.
5. **Golden milk**: In a saucepan combine 1 cup of milk or non- dairy alternative with ½ teaspoon of ground turmeric, ¼ teaspoon of cinnamon, ¼ teaspoon of ground ginger and a pinch of black pepper. Optionally you can add a drizzle of honey.
6. **Yerba mate**: Leave the leaves (using a tea ball) or a yerba mate tea bag in hot water for 3-5 mins.
7. **Chai tea**: In a pot, combine ½ cup of milk or non-dairy alternative and ½ cup of water with 2 green cardamom pods, ½ teaspoon of ground cinnamon, 1 black tea bag and 2 slices of ginger. Leave on

the lowest heat setting for 7-10 mins, then strain into a cup, add a drizzle of honey and enjoy. If you just want to add water and milk and have a chai latte powder mix ready this is my favourite one: Pukka Majestic Matcha Chai Latte.

8. **Rooibos tea**: Use a tea filter to steep 1-1.5 teaspoons of loose rooibos for up to 10 mins or use a rooibos tea bag and leave in hot water for 2-3 mins.

9. **Kombucha tea**: Making Kombucha on your own is not recommended, so here my favourite one: Ginger Lemon Kombucha from Remedy Company.

10. **Peppermint tea**: Use 7-10 leaves or 1 tea bag in 250ml of hot water and let steep for 2 mins.

Chapter Four
Dear Stress

I have to be perfect…

I am frustrated…

I am not good enough…

I have relationship problems…

I am trying to please everybody…

I am scare of failing…...

I am always comparing myself to others….

I have financial problems…

I am suffering from burnout…

My life is full of hassle…

I am suffering from illness…

Someone close to me has passed away…

All you need to do is to learn to forecast your stress levels. In today's world everything has to be done so fast that you end up burnt out and drained of energy at the end of the day. In the graph below you can see how stress vs performance works. We want to be in the rockin' it! stage. In this chapter you will learn to identify how much stress you have and how to maintain a middle point stress level during the day.

Stress Vs Performance

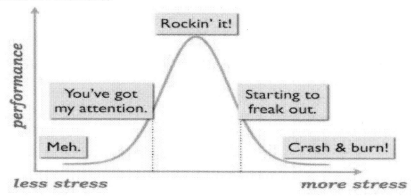

Stress Awareness Questionnaire

- Do you sleep less than 6 hours per night? ☐ Yes ☐ No

- Do you have trouble falling asleep? ☐ Yes ☐ No

- Do you feel like you have incomplete sleep? ☐ Yes ☐ No

- Do you feel tired but wired? ☐ Yes ☐ No

- Do you have a midday crash in energy? ☐ Yes ☐ No

- Do you have dark circles under your eyes? ☐ Yes ☐ No

- Do you crave sugars or carbs in the afternoon and evening? ☐ Yes ☐ No

- Do you feel anxious or nervous? ☐ Yes ☐ No

- Are you easily irritated or get grumpy easily with family or colleagues? ☐ Yes ☐ No

- Are you under high stress/overcommitted personally or at work? ☐ Yes ☐ No

What happens when stress is too much?

High blood pressure   Hunger (cravings)

Low sex drive

Delayed recovery

Water retention

Mood swings and anxiety

Lowered emotional state

Muscle loss   Poor sleep

Weakened immune system

Lowered energy levels   Increased fat storage   Irregular menstrual cycle

Stress and fitness

Stress control can – and should – involve the body. Aerobic exercise is one approach.

The relaxed body will send signals of calm and control that help reduce mental tension.

You should exercise nearly every day. That does not necessarily mean hitting the gym, 30 to 40 minutes of moderate exercise such as walking, or 15 to 20 minutes of vigorous exercise is enough.

How exercise reduces stress

In the beginning, exercise will be more work than fun but as you get into shape, you will begin to tolerate exercise, then enjoy it and finally depend on it. Regular aerobic exercise will bring remarkable changes to your body, your metabolism, your heart and your spirit.

Exercise reduces the levels of the body's stress hormones, such as adrenaline and cortisol. It also stimulates the production of endorphins, chemicals in the brain that are the body's natural painkillers and mood elevators. Endorphins are responsible for the feelings of relaxation and optimism that accompany many hard workouts – or, at least, the hot shower after your exercise is over.

As your waistline shrinks, your self-image will improve. You will feel pride in your achievements and self-confidence and the discipline of regular exercise will help you achieve other important lifestyle goals. Almost any type of exercise activity will help.

How to breathe while exercising

The best advice I can give you is simple, smile while you are training!

Ideas to prevent/manage stress and recovery

- Warm drink breaks during the day: 5 mins
- Bath with relaxing salts e.g. Epsom: 15-30 mins
- Sauna: 30- 60 mins
- Massage or self-massage: 5-30 mins
- Yoga/Pilates: 5-30 mins
- Take a nap: 10-30 mins
- Rest days: no activity at all, just walks
- Exercise: 15-30 mins, 3-4 times per week
- Essential oils: lavender or peppermint
- Reduce caffeine intake: 3 to 4 cups per day
- Write things down: any thoughts such as ideas or things to do
- Spend time with friends/family: after work/studies or a full day, it can be face to face or by video call
- Laugh: funny videos on YouTube
- Avoid procrastination: have only 2-3 priorities per day
- Practice meditation: 5-10 minutes guided meditation on YouTube or a mobile app like Calm
- Cuddle: find someone for a short/long cuddle or a self-cuddle is great too
- Listen to music: create a playlist with your favourite songs
- Deep breathing: 5 deep breaths a few times a day
- Spend time with your pet: go for a walk with your dog
- Dance: watch a zumba or hip-hop choreography
- Watch a funny video: cat or babies are the best ones
- Practice gratitude: write 5-10 things you are grateful for

The Mindset checklist: prevent and manage stress

Checklist stress management	M	T	W	T	F	S	S	Comments or changes
Spend time with friends and family			☑	☑				Videocall better than call
Dance		☑						Awesome, got new friends
Meditation	☑				☑			Morning 5 mins, feel great
Laugh	☑		☑	☑				10 mins James Corden
Avoid Procrastination			☑		☑	☑		To do list works great
Exercise				☑	☑			Increase exercise to 3 times a week for 30 mins each day.
Reduce caffeine intake	☑	☑	☑	☑	☑	☑	☑	No later than 3 pm
Essential oil	☑							Before bed
Bed Tea					☑			Makes me sleepy, avoid, find a new one
Bath	☑				☑			Works well just for 30 mins

Having this weekly report with you will allow you to forecast a burnout and help to take control of your daily performance, because what usually happens is that we learn to take action once we have the problem in front of us, not before it happens.

This checklist is really simple. Choose and write down your favourites ideas to prevent/manage stress and recovery for your week and then tick off which days you did it and add any comments or changes for the following week.

Now it's time for you to practice:

The Mindset checklist template – prevent and manage stress

Checklist stress management	M	T	W	T	F	S	S	Comments or changes

Chapter Five
Sleep for Fat Loss

Sleep is essential for fat loss and getting less of it means your nutrition plan may be destined to end in snacking all day long and not making the right decisions to win the day. 'A good night's sleep will magnify your training and nutrition. A bad night's sleep will serve as a hormonal handbrake to your fat loss,' says Ross Edgley in *The World's Fittest Book*.

Sleep Hygiene Questionnaire

- Do you sleep in a room with any light or noise? ☐ Yes ☐ No

- Do you wake up feeling tired? ☐ Yes ☐ No

- Do you go to bed later than 11 p.m.? ☐ Yes ☐ No

- Do you struggle to fall asleep? ☐ Yes ☐ No

- Do you get up earlier than 6 a.m.? ☐ Yes ☐ No

- Do you use medications to help you sleep? ☐ Yes ☐ No

Why do we need sleep?

- Performance and recovery for the day ahead
- Managing blood sugar
- Immune health/limit inflammation
- Optimal metabolic function
- Rejuvenates the brain
- Muscle recovery
- Improved cognitive function
- Sleep deprivation has been linked to insulin resistance, weight gain and depression

Sleep Quality and Duration Questionnaire

- Do you have trouble falling asleep at night?   ☐ Yes   ☐ No

- Do you have difficulty waking up in the morning?   ☐ Yes   ☐ No

- Do you sleep less than 7-8 hours a night?   ☐ Yes   ☐ No

- Do you wake up once or more in the night?   ☐ Yes   ☐ No

- If you do wake up, what time is it at?

  ☐ 1-3 a.m.   ☐ 3-5 a.m.   ☐ Wake up tired at 5 a.m.   ☐ Many times, throughout the night

In the case study below, you will see the importance of 6-8 hours of quality sleep a day to improve fat loss results. If you sleep less than 6 hours in bed it will be harder to see results. The below graph is taken from *The World's Fittest Book* by Ross Edgley.

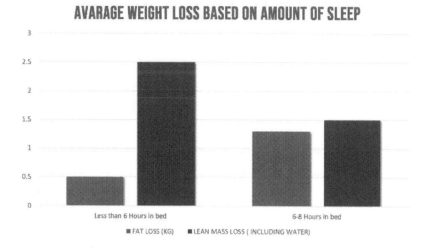

AVARAGE WEIGHT LOSS BASED ON AMOUNT OF SLEEP

Improving your sleep quality

1. **Sleep in a dark room (complete blackout)** making sure you have an *eye mask and earplugs.* This will help you get more quality rest and recovery.

2. **Manage stimulant intake (supplements)**. If you love having a cup of coffee, tea or an energy drink – this totally fine, we all like it – in my personal opinion, and what works for me, is to reduce caffeine *before 6 p.m. if possible.*
   Note: Caffeine can stay in your body for more than two hours, but this will depend on your caffeine sensitivity.

3. **Create sleep habits (evening routine)**. Taking some time to think about what you do, what you would like to do and what you need to do before bed will allow you to *create awareness and improve rest and recovery* while you are sleeping.

4. **Maintain a healthy blood sugar balance**. This will be linked with the *type, quality and variety of nutrients in your daily intake*. For example, adding beans, fruit, vegetables, fish or water and creating a balance and moderation of the food that you like.
   Example: Having pasta with chicken in tomato sauce and parmesan cheese on top.
   Better option: Having pasta with chicken in *natural* tomato sauce and a sprinkle of parmesan cheese on top with a salad of lettuce and cucumber on the side.

5. **Manage screen time, or limit exposure to blue light**. Nowadays our phone is our second hand, we cannot live without it, however making sure you have a blue light filter app or set a timer on your phone to activate bedtime mode is a great help.
   Example: You could activate this app around 8:30 p.m. till 6 a.m.

6. **Maintain a room temperature of around 18-22 degrees celsius**. Keeping a nice cool room has been proved to aid optimal sleep and recovery, due to our bodies being at the lowest body temperature and blood pressure according to sleep cycle research.

7. **Do not take the bedroom as a centre for entertainment (TV, books, etc. should be in the living room)**. This a hard one to follow because sometimes we like to watch TV, read or use our phone in bed. It is beneficial to limit the use of those devices or items 2 hours before bedtime, if possible.

8. **Working out** is an important component of having a restful sleep.

Make sure to do some physical activity, or at least go for walk, and aim to have a productive day, where your body will be active.

9. **Taking a nap** is a great tool for people who are early birds or just like to have a short rest during a long day. The amount recommended by experts, and from my personal experience, is between 15 to 30 mins max between 1 and 3 p.m.

Sleep is not always complicated. It is about using every single tool we have to make it possible to rest and recover every night.

Supplements to support sleep and aid recovery

I know how frustrating it can be not being able to have a restful sleep and for that reason I will share with you the best supplements to improve sleep and recovery:

- **Magnesium glycinate** is a key nutrient for our bodies playing an important role in our health, notably for our brain, heart and muscles. There is no ideal dose because it will vary from person to person, however a good starting point is 250-500mg to see how your body assimilates it. I recommend Magnesium Glycinate because it has very good absorption levels meaning your body can make the most of it once it's ingested.
- **Melatonin** is natural hormone that your body produces in the pineal gland which then sends signals to the brain, eyes, bone marrow and gut. Nevertheless, melatonin will not be a sleep miracle for you. It works as an alarm that will let you know that it is time to wind down, so you fall asleep easier. The recommended dosage is 2-5 mg per day.
- **L-theanine** will improve quality of sleep, lower anxiety and will

increase relaxation. You can find this amino acid in tea leaves for example, green or black tea and also in supplements. If you are taking a pill or tablet, the recommended dosage is 300 mg per day.

- **Ashwagandha** is an organic sleep aid that will allow you to deal with insomnia and improve sleep quality. The recommended dosage is 500-1000 mg split through the day or 2 hours before bed.

Why do we have to create an evening routine?

An evening routine can help expedite and streamline your mornings. Part of an evening routine is to start doing things in the evening so you can save time in the morning.

- What you don't do in your evening routine, will affect your morning routine.
- An evening routine will help you ensure you go to bed on time so that you can wake up on time.
- The evening routine is what sets you up for success.
- You'll get plenty of restorative sleep, feel great when you wake up and be able to use your time strategically in the morning!
- If you've ever felt like your morning was stressful, chances are it is because you didn't have a plan.

Write your own evening routine in six steps

1. **Figure out what time you need to go to bed**: We need to work backwards to build out your evening routine. For example, if you want to wake up at 5 a.m. and need 7.5 hours of sleep, that means you need to be asleep (not in bed, but asleep!) by 9:30 p.m. to get enough sleep.

2. **Review your list of evening tasks**: Identify several tasks that you do in the evening. For example, walk the dog, time with family/friends, social media, etc.

3. **Add things to the list that will help you have a more productive morning**: What could you do before bed to be more productive the next day? For example, set up breakfast the night before or maybe you need to plan out your to do list for the day. Anything that comes to mind, add it to the list.

4. **Add to the list things you *want* to do in the evenings**: For example, maybe you want to read for 30 minutes or maybe you want to learn how to cook. Whatever it is, add it all to your list!

5. **Estimate how long each task will take**: Look at your list and decide how long each of these things is going to take you. Go line by line and determine a timescale for each item on your list. For example:

    a. Walk the dog – 30 mins

    b. Social media – 1 hour

    c. Preset up breakfast – 15 mins

    d. Read a book – 30 mins

You will find the sweet spot for you with time.

My daily mindset evening routine example:

Date:		Total time for routine: 2h 15 mins approx.		
Times backwards	To do routine	Check here ☑		Comments or changes
11:30 – 11:10 pm	Go to bed	Yes ☑ No		
11:30 – 11:10 pm	Read (optional), pray	Yes No ☑		I'd rather read in the afternoon.
11:10 – 11 pm	Bed tea time	Yes No ☑		Having a tea was not for me. Will try a small glass of milk instead.
11 – 10:45 pm	Prepare bag and clothes for tomorrow	Yes ☑ No		
10:45 – 10:30 pm	Personal hygiene	Yes ☑ No		15 mins is an ideal time.
10:30 – 10:15 pm	Food prep for next day	Yes No		
10:15 – 10 pm	(last check), put phone airplane mode	Yes ☑ No		
10 – 9:30 pm	Commute to home	Yes No ☑		I will cycle to skip the traffic jam and have more time to do something else.
9:30 – 9:15 pm	Get ready to go home	Yes ☑ No		
9:15 – 9 pm	Plan to do list for tomorrow	Yes ☑ No		

Your mindset evening routine template

Step one: Put a date and the total time you will spend approximately

Step two: Write your evening list activities down

Step three: Check in by ticking the Yes or No box

Step four: Add any comments or changes for the next day

Date:	Times backwards	To do routine	Check here	Total time for routine:	Comments or changes
			Yes ☐ No ☐		
			Yes ☐ No ☐		
			Yes ☐ No ☐		
			Yes ☐ No ☐		
			Yes ☐ No ☐		
			Yes ☐ No ☐		
			Yes ☐ No ☐		
			Yes ☐ No ☐		
			Yes ☐ No ☐		
			Yes ☐ No ☐		

32

The Circadian sleep pattern

As you can see in the graphic below, the quality of your sleep pattern is linked with your cortisol levels and how you manage your stress. Nowadays in society we think that stress is bad for us, but it's not. Usually in a person who has a good quality of sleep, cortisol levels will rise at the beginning of the day and naturally will decrease at the end of the day.

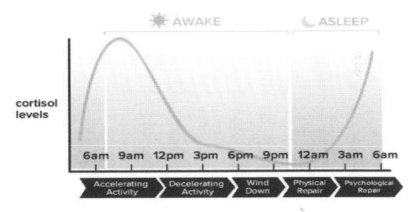

My personal opinion and advice to you

If you want to improve your sleep quality you need to make sure to wind down from any external stimulant around 8 p.m., if possible. This will allow you to have a good quality night's sleep. If you are still reading emails, not switching off from work and watching tv, especially the news or videos, or listening to music or reading things that will keep stimulating your brain such as horror or action, you won't be able to sleep properly.

Instead, try to aim to wind down with a nice bath, reading a motivational book or watching something on TV or Netflix with an inspirational message or a comedy movie or having a self-massage.

To summarise, you need to keep your stress levels in control during the day because this will allow you to perform your best, but aim to reduce activities and complex tasks after 6 p.m.

Chapter Six

Bye Bad Digestion

It is not just about what we eat, but, more importantly, how we absorb what we eat. If you have poor digestion, fat loss and gaining muscle tissue will be really challenging.

It is a long process for your stomach to fully recover and can take up to 18 months.
To have an idea of how fragile your stomach lining is, put one finger on the back of your eyelid and feel how soft and sensitive the skin is there.

For that reason, we need to take into consideration what is making us bloated. Just as when you roll your ankle and it immediately swells up, every time you get bloated your immune system is triggered by responding with a pump of fluid and cytokines into the area. Therefore, it is important to avoid being constantly bloated.

Inflammation will be the link to fat gain.

Other associated signs of digestive dysfunction:
  - Depression, anxiety and mood changes
  - Joint pain
  - Acne
  - Asthma and allergies
  - Migraines
  - Fatigue
  - Frequent illness and infections

- Frequent blood sugar fluctuations throughout the day
- Sinus issues

Digestive System Questionnaire:

- Do you suffer from indigestion or heart burn? ☐ Yes ☐ No
- Do you suffer from gas or belching? ☐ Yes ☐ No
- Do you suffer from constipation? ☐ Yes ☐ No
- Do you suffer from diarrhea? ☐ Yes ☐ No
- Do you have a sense of fullness after your meals? ☐ Yes ☐ No
- Do you suffer from bloating 1 hour after eating? ☐ Yes ☐ No
- Do you suffer from bad breath? ☐ Yes ☐ No

The role of the digestive system

- Sterilises food
- Breaks food down
- Protects us from infection
- Disposes of toxins
- Determines which nutrients to absorb
- Determines which toxins to clear out

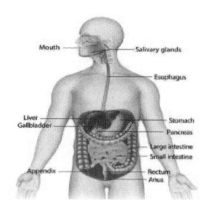

Why you may have an unhealthy digestive system

Do you have a too-full feeling in the belly after you eat a bit too much? Or it might be the type of food you ate or how fast you ate it. It could be too much salt, fat or sugar. All these things cause gas, bloating, weight gain, constipation or water retention.

Foods that may trigger digestive issues:

- **Fried foods**: These are high in saturated fats and trans fats which make them extremely low in fiber and nutrients therefore you may experience diarrhea, bloating or constipation.
- **Citrus fruits**: Some people may get an upset stomach because citruses like lemons or oranges are high in acid.
- **Artificial sugar**: If you like to chew sugar-free gums make sure to check if they contain sorbitol, because you may get cramps and diarrhea.
- **Fibre**: If you suddenly start eating more vegetables, salads or beans than you used to do, you may have some issues with gas and bloating due to your digestive system needing to adjust to it. So, make sure to increase the portion of fibre in your day-to-day diet in a progressive amount until you find the desired amount that works for you.
- **Beans and legumes**: Some people may not have the digestive enzymes to break down these complex sugars. Also, their high amount of fibre may cause gas and cramping.
- **Fructose**: Nowadays we have two types of fructose: the organic type found in vegetables, honey and fruits which you can include as part of your balanced nutrition and the manufactured HFCS found in soft drinks, sweets, fruit juices or pastries which may lead

to diarrhea, bloating and cramps because some people find it difficult to digest.

- **Cruciferous vegetables like broccoli and cabbage:** If you experience some digestive issues such as gas, make sure to cook these instead of eating them raw.
- **Spicy foods**: Most of us love it, however you may experience indigestion or heartburn, mainly after eating a large meal. Reduce the amount you're eating and to prevent any of those symptoms, warm-up your digestive system with some dairy before any meal such as a full tablespoon of yogurt which will neutralise the effect.
- **Dairy products**: I've recommended dairy to prevent side effects from spicy food, however you may get diarrhea, bloating or gas because of lactose intolerance which means you do not have a digestive enzyme that digests sugar in milk and other forms of dairy.
- **Peppermint tea, chocolate or coffee**: It may relax the upper part of your stomach letting acid go through the esophagus causing you heartburn.

If you experience digestive issues, I suggest losing any extra weight, eating an ideal portion for you and avoiding lying down after eating. It is also useful to learn which foods give you problems so you can avoid them.

Supplements to support digestion:
- **Digestive enzymes** – 1-2 tablets with each meal
- **Probiotics** – these add good bacteria and boost the immune system. 2 capsules a day with food and find a probiotic that works for you

- **Fish oil** – Ideal for inflammation. 1 capsule per day (1000 mg 180EPA/120DHA)
- **Zinc** – 25 mg per day
- **Glutamine** – 5-10 g per day spread out
- **Apple cider vinegar** – 1 teaspoon, one to two times per day (15-20 mins before meals)
- **Aloe Vera juice** – 1 shot in the morning and 1 shot in the evening
- **Turmeric and black pepper** – 1 capsule a day

Natural supplements to support digestion:
- **Ginger**: Eating or drinking foods with ginger will promote contractions in the muscles that line the digestive organs.
- **Miso**: Made of fermented soya beans, miso is a rich source of digestive enzymes and a good source of probiotics.
- **Pineapple**: Eating pineapple alongside protein-rich foods supports digestion of the meal. Try baked pineapple with cinnamon as a dessert.
- **Kimchi**: Originally from Korea, kimchi has bacteria that produce digestive enzymes that are good for your body overall.
- **Mango**: They are rich in enzymes and fibre allowing you to break down protein content in your body.
- **Papaya**: Eat it raw, so you get the most benefit from the papain enzymes which help better digestion.
- **Avocado**: These are rich in enzymes and fibre which may help prevent the uncomfortable 'full' feeling after a meal and avoid constipation.
- **Apricots**: Great source of vitamins A, C and E and iron. Apricots can also help to ease constipation, acid reflux and indigestion.

- **Banana**: They have a good dose of digestive enzymes. To get the best benefits from bananas eat them when they are all yellow with brown flecks.
- **Kiwi**: Contains a digestive enzyme called actinidin that helps break down protein, helping you with constipation and bloating.
- **Water:** Drink 2-3 litres of water per day. Hydration is key for bowel movements.

Practice Time
- Identify your food trigger
- Write your food trigger digestive checklist

The Mindset food trigger digestive checklist – example:
This daily or weekly chart will allow you to identify food triggers and which symptoms you are experiencing and will help you to develop awareness in your body.

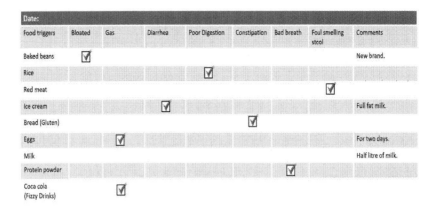

Date:								
Food triggers	Bloated	Gas	Diarrhea	Poor Digestion	Constipation	Bad breath	Foul smelling stool	Comments
Baked beans	☑							New brand.
Rice				☑				
Red meat							☑	
Ice cream			☑					Full fat milk.
Bread (Gluten)					☑			
Eggs		☑						For two days.
Milk								Half litre of milk.
Protein powder							☑	
Coca cola (Fizzy Drinks)		☑						

My Mindset food trigger digestive checklist – template:

Step one: Put the full date or start to end date.

Step two: Write any new potential or old food triggers you think you may have.

Step three: Cross with an X any symptoms you may have with food trigger/s and add any comments that will help you create more awareness, such as ingredients, how long you have been using it for or even the time of the day you had it.

Date:	Food triggers	Bloated	Gas	Diarrhea	Poor Digestion	Constipation	Bad breath	Foul smelling stool	Comments

Nowadays, in our society, we have supermarkets and food available to us anywhere we go, but a long time ago it was a long process to obtain food or even prepare it, when it was necessary to cultivate and hunt our food.

Anticipation of our food is one of the most important tools we have. The more time we take to think, prepare and care about what we are going to eat, the greater the increase of salivation which will help us to take in food and nutrients more efficiently because we are sending signals to our digestive system to get ready for food coming up.

For our ancestors, meal preparation was a ritual, something special.
Is food a ritual for you?

Chapter Seven
Healthy Vs Junk Food

Do you feel like a failure if you eat a cookie or an ice cream?

When I started my fitness journey, I believed that to be in shape and to achieve your fitness goals you must only eat 'healthy food' every day for the rest of your life.

I have been, and still am, fighting with this belief and teaching my athletes that it is okay to have an ice cream or to have cookies if you want. As long as 80 per cent of your nutrition is coming from whole food (Mother Earth), it is fine to have something every day you believe is not 'healthy.'

What I usually do once a month, or once in a while, or on special occasions, is to have a day off completely and I will eat whatever I like. Yes, it might seem crazy, but nothing will happen as long you are back on track the next day, week, month and year, because you are working to improve and maintain long-term goals for life not just for a short period of time.

So, next time you feel anxious about having pizza, burgers, cookies or ice cream, enjoy it and then be back on track with your fitness routine, your training plan, nutrition plan and your fitness goals.

Be kind to yourself – extreme is not a good place to be, harmony is the best option.

Chapter Eight
The Real Fat Loss Supplements

With many supplements on the market, you may feel confused about which are the best to optimize your fitness journey. Here is a summary of the supplements I recommend:

Primary supplements (essential ones):

1. Fish oil: Fish oil helps to fight inflammation in our body which can lead to being overweight and having health issues.
Benefits: Improves endurance, builds muscle, helps you perform better, improves reaction time, burns fat and aids faster recovery.

Action plan: Take one capsule a day of 1000 mg (EPA 180MG, DHA 120MG)

2. Complex B: This gives us more energy, helping to reduce stress by supporting the nervous system. It supports the digestive system to break down food more easily thus converting it to fuel (energy).
Benefits: Increases energy, enhances mood, improves memory, boosts skin and hair health, stimulates the immune system, forms red blood cells.

Action plan: Take one tablet a day with plenty of liquid.

3. Multivitamins: If you find you don't have enough variety of fruit and vegetables you might consider having this supplement next to you. It contains additional nutrients that you might not find in your own fruit and vegetable intake.

Note: Nutrients you find in fruit and veg are key for our health. They shore up bones, heal wounds and bolster your immune system. They also convert food into energy and repair cellular damage.

Action plan: Take one tablet a day with plenty of liquid.

4. Sleep aids: Getting quality sleep is really important for fat loss. If you find it difficult to sleep, use natural supplements to help you decrease cortisol levels, which are linked with levels of stress during the day, and you will have better control of your hunger and cravings. You will recover faster and will have more energy during the day. For that reason, it is really important to have a good quality and quantity of sleep every day.

Action plan: Take one tablet of 250mg of magnesium or ashwagandha or a small cup of warm chamomile or milk 1 to 2 hours before bed. This will allow you to have a wonderful sleep.

5. Vitamin D: If you are living in a European country like me, you will know that we don't have sunlight 24 hours per day, 365 days per year, and for that reason it is really important to supplement ourselves with vitamin D. Why? Having some sunlight in our body is essential for bones, blood cells and your immune system.

Action plan: Make sure you have one large egg per day which is equivalent to 41 units of vitamin D or take one tablet which contributes

50 units per day.

Extra supplements (non-essential ones):

1. Protein powder: Use this supplement when you find yourself having difficulty eating meat or any protein source. This is when protein powder becomes useful. Covering our protein requirements per day is really important. It will allow us to recover our muscles as well as grow more muscle, result in us having more muscle rather than body fat.

Note: If you can cover your daily protein intake make sure you eat whole food such as meat, beans, fish and eggs.

Action plan: 2 scoops of 30g (each scoop) per day as maximum intake.

2. Caffeine: Feeling energised after a cup of coffee or tea is great and there is nothing wrong with it. It will allow us to push a bit more in our workouts, work and studies, or it might be just because we love the taste and the aroma of the coffee.

Action plan: Enjoy any caffeine beverage until 5/6 p.m. in the evening. Also make sure to limit to four cups of coffee, tea or two cans of energy drinks per day.

3. Green mixed vegetable powder: Not a big fan of vegetables? Especially green vegetables? That's fine because nowadays everything is possible, you can have your green vegetables every day with no problem at all. This supplement is even sweet, has no taste of vegetables and is really yummy. The process of micro-pulverisation in this powder makes it possible to cover our daily intake of vitamins and minerals that we get from those green vegetables.

Action plan: One serving of 5g per day with plenty of liquid.

Remember, in order to achieve fat loss results we need to have a 360-degree approach. This means your training, nutrition, sleep, stress and digestion need to be on top. Combine this with empowering yourself with those supplements and you will become unstoppable.

Chapter Nine

How to Create Fat Loss SMART Goals

How about if I tell you that with this SMART formula you can achieve and keep your fitness results for the long term, without stressing yourself out.

Let's crack on!

S: This letter stands for specific

Here you need to think about the goal you want to achieve but you need to be as *specific as possible*.

Example: I want to lose as much body weight as I can.

Specific **Example**: I want to lose *5 kgs* of body weight.

My Specific example is/are:

-

-

-

M: Measurable:

Which *actions* will you take in order to achieve your goal?

Example: I will work out 3 times a week.

Measurable **Example**:

- I will work out 3 times a week for 60 mins each session.

- I will have 3 main meals of 500 calories each meal in order to create a caloric deficit and therefore lose weight.

- I will walk for 15 mins every day.

- I will track my training plan and nutrition plan every week/month

Note: the more actions and tools you have the better the results.

My Measurable example is/are:
A: Attainable
Do you feel that even though it will be challenging, it will be possible *to achieve this goal*?
Example:
-I will work out 3 times a week for 60 mins plus a 30 mins HIIT workout each session -I will cut down on bread, sugar and chocolate from my nutritional lifestyle
-I will eat just salad until I lose 5 kg of body weight

Attainable **Example**:
- I will work out 3 times a week for 60 mins and monthly I will have *one* HIIT training of *10 mins each session* and then *slowly increase* the total amount of this HIIT workout.
- I will *moderate my portion*s of bread, sugar and chocolate during a day-to-day basis.
- I will make sure I have all my nutrients in my meals and have a weight loss *nutrition plan* that will allow me to keep seeing results without *starving myself.*

My Attainable example is/are:
-

-

-

R: Relevant
Your goals should align with your *values* and *long-term objectives*.
Example:
- I will change my nutrition lifestyle just for my holidays/wedding
- I want to get ready for summer and then come back to my normal (old) habits.

Relevant Example:
- I will change my nutrition lifestyle because I want to be *healthy and energetic every day.*
- I want to change my lifestyle because I want to *look great physically and be healthy all year round.*

My Relevant example is/are:
-

-

-

T: Time-Based

When is a *realistic deadline* to achieve this goal?

Example: I want to lose 5kg of body weight in 2 weeks.

***Time-Based* Example**: I will lose 5kg of body weight in *4-8 weeks' time*.

My Time-based example is/are:

-

-

-

Remember:

WE ALL WORK EFFECTIVE WHEN WE HAVE GOALS TO GO AFTER.

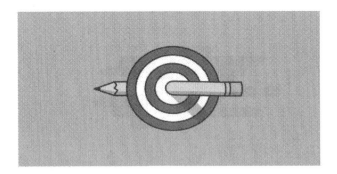

NO GOAL IS IMPOSSIBLE, JUST HAVE A GOOD PLAN TO WORK WITH

Chapter Ten

The Power of Small Wins

What do small wins mean to you? Are they important to you?

Have you seen yourself in the mirror? Sometimes we blind ourselves just waiting to see results on the scale, but you need to see your performance in your daily activity.

- If you have more energy than before...
- If you feel happier than before...
- If you feel more confident than before...
- If you have received compliments recently on how slim/fit, you are...
- If you see yourself wanting to work out more often...
- If you are caring about your nutrition...
- If you see that your clothes do not fit anymore...
      ...all of these are small wins.

Action Plan: Next time you feel frustrated about not seeing results, sit down and write five small wins you have accomplished since the beginning of your fitness journey and try to improve these in the following 4 weeks.

My five small wins are...

First small win:

Second small win:

Third small win:

Fourth small win:

Fifth small win:

Conclusion
How to be Motivated for Life

I will inspire you and share with you my 5 biggest reasons to be motivated for life:

1. Family medical history: I don't want to have diabetes, most of my family are likely to have it. Being aware of this allows me to think that I need to take action today rather than tomorrow when it might be too late. Remembering my grandmother injecting insulin every day is a big incentive to do everything I can in order to take care of myself today.
Note: Sometimes you can use your fears as a strength that will allow you to be consistent with what you do.

2. Fitness dad: My dad is my example. After brain surgery and with half of his body paralysed, he is still doing, almost every day, his recovery exercises with a strong belief that he will recover. Believe it or not, he increased his mobility by 50 per cent in one year after his surgery.
Note: Try to think about someone who inspires you. It doesn't matter if they are real or not, just have someone who will fire you up and motivate you to be like him/her.

3. Example of my family: Many of my family members are overweight. Growing up in a house where there was not a good relationship with food made me understand myself in a better way and motivated me to try to help myself and the people around me at the same time. To be honest it is something that I am really grateful for.
Note: Take a decision today and promise yourself you will be the

example for your family and show them that it is possible to be fit, healthy and, most importantly, have a good relationship with food and enjoy life.

4. Change the meaning of elderly: Visualising myself at 70 years old, I want to be working on my well-being, being able to travel anywhere, climbing or cycling with my grandchildren, doing any physical activity and, most importantly, not depending on any medication or spending hours or even days at the hospital. How would you like to live life when you're 70 years old?

5. Childhood memories: For a good period of my childhood, I was overweight. I was not happy about other people calling me by nicknames rather than my name, I didn't trust myself and I was worried about how I looked and what other people thought about me. But nowadays I am happy about where and how I am and having a fitness plan helps so much with my confidence and to keep on track too.

Note*: Build a fitness plan and use any downsides in your life to empower yourself and become your best version of you.*

Remember: Having and being aware of your 5 biggest reasons will help you become more inspired and motivated to do it, even if you don't feel like it.

So, what are your 5 biggest reason to be motivated for life?

Reason 1:

Reason 2:

Reason 3:

Reason 4:

Reason 5:

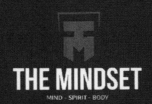

THE MINDSET
MIND - SPIRIT - BODY

LOVE:
Universal love is an expression of the harmony of everything
and everyone in the universe.
You are a part of everything; each person you know and each person
you meet is connected to one another.
We are all spiritual beings in human form with an abundance of love,
energy, and knowledge that is universal.

SERVICE:
The soul is motivated by service.
Being a tool of service is what makes us the happiest and most fulfilled.
Serve yourself, serve the people, serve the community, serve the universe.
Be a selfless soul that leaves a mark in the world.

IMPROVE:
Don't live life being the world's version of you.
Become the person you want to be, step by step, one day at a time.
Be better than you were yesterday, just 1%. That's all it takes.

Hope you can achive everything you put into this book, these ideas and thoughts
are yours, they can be true as long as you do your best to make them happen,
remember everything you write down here matters, there are
emotions and feelings in every word, believe in
yourself because I believe in you!

Love, Serve and Improve every day.

The Mindset Family.

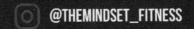 @THEMINDSET_FITNESS

Exercise Library

Warm up examples

Neck and shoulder circles

A: Stand straight with your arms by your sides and with your feet shoulder width apart.

B: Tilt your head to the left

C: Start rolling head and shoulder at the same time, making big circles until the set time is complete

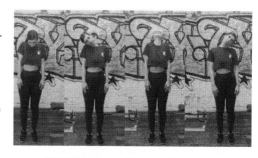

Angel walls

A: Stand tall with your feet shoulder width apart and position your arms at a 70-degree angle

B: Make sure hands are in line with your shoulders

C: Extend arms fully towards the ceiling

D: Repeat the process

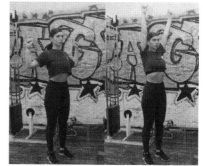

Cow and cat

A: Begin by kneeling on hands and knees

B: Position hands shoulder width apart and knees hip distance apart

C: Inhale and look up to the ceiling, arching your back

D: Exhale and curve your back towards the ceiling, like an angry cat, and look towards your knees

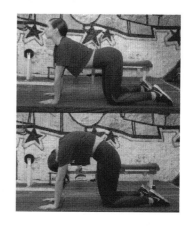

Training Program

Legs Compound Muscle Group Examples

Hip raises

A: Lie on your back with your knees bent and your arms down by your sides

B: Press firmly through your feet and engage your glutes to lift up the hips, creating a straight line from the heels to the shoulders

C: Hold for two seconds and lower slowly

D: Repeat

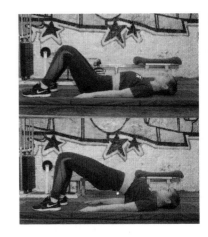

Squats and lunges

A: Stand with your feet shoulder width apart

B: Bend at your hips and knees to lower yourself into a squatting position

C: Bring yourself back to standing, and with one leg, step backward

D: Flex your knees and lower your hips, until the back knee is just above the floor

E: Return to the standing position to then bring the other leg backward

F: Start again from the top

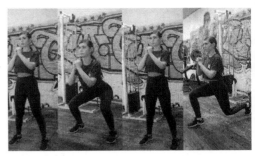

Back Compound Muscle Group Examples

Bird dog

A: Begin in a quadruped position with your core engaged

B: Slowly raise one arm and the opposite leg to torso height

C: Your hips and shoulders should continue facing the floor

D: Slowly lower and repeat the same process on each side until the set time is complete

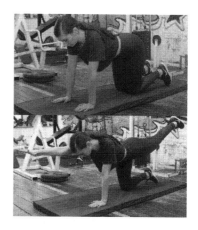

Superman

A: Lie on your belly, with your arms and legs fully extended

B: Raise both arms off the floor and hold for 2 seconds

C: Return to the starting position and repeat

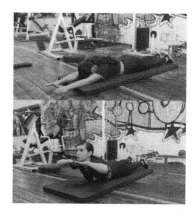

Chest Compound Muscle Group Examples

Wider push ups

A: Position your body in a straight line with your arms fully extended, shoulder width apart, core tight

B: Lower your body until your chest almost reaches the floor, keeping elbows straight on your way down

C: Push your torso away from the floor until your arms lock

D: Repeat

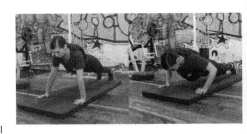

MMA Push ups

A: Position your body in a straight line with your arms fully extended. For the close push ups keep both hands as close as possible to each other, for the medium push ups keep hands shoulder width apart and for the wider push ups keep hands more open than shoulder width apart. For each push up, keep the core tight

B: Lower your body until your chest almost reaches the floor, keep elbows straight on your way down

C: Push your torso away from the floor until your arms lock

D: Repeat the same process for each push up

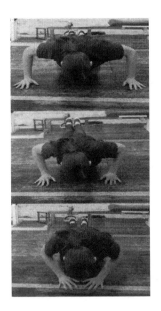

Core Isolation Muscle Group Example

Sit up punches

A: Lie on your back, keep knees bent and feet flat on the floor

B: Keep core tight, sit up and punch across your body as fast as you can for 4 seconds with both arms

C: Repeat the process

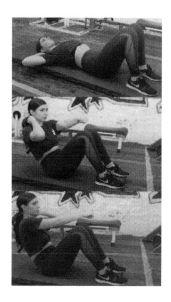

Cardiovascular Exercise Example

Quiet burpee

A: Stand with your feet shoulder width apart

B: Bend at your hips and knees to lower yourself into a squatting position and touch the floor with your hands

C: Walk your feet back so your body is in a straight line

D: Stand up by walking your feet forward, then repeat the process

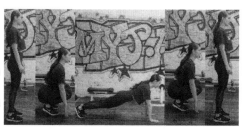

Cool Down Examples

Auto hug

A: Lie down on your back and pull both knees up to your chest

B: Slowly pull your knees toward your shoulders until you feel the stretch in your lower back

C: Stay in this position for 30 seconds

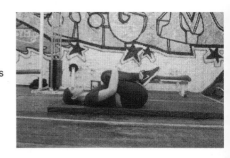

Knee to chest

A: Lie on your back with your legs extended in front of you and with the backs of your heels on the floor

B: Grab your right knee and gently pull it up as close as you can to your chest while keeping the left leg relaxed

C: Hold the stretch for 15 seconds and then release the leg to starting position

D: Repeat with the left leg for 15 seconds

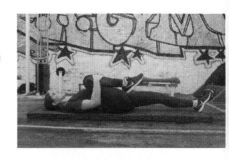

Kneeling back

A: Be on your hands and knees, walk your right hand forward and slide the left hand between the right knee and the right hand

B: Twist your torso to the left and rest your head on your mat

C: Stay in this position for 15 seconds, return to neutral position, then reverse hands and repeat the process on the other side for 15 seconds

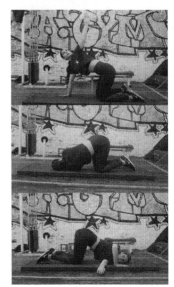

Online Bonus

Links to YouTube exercises ideas and nutritional guidelines.

Exercise Examples:

TMS Warm Up YouTube Playlist:

https://www.youtube.com/playlist?list=PLYIhIvKYrLX6GxDeTErtXe5tdq8GINqrB

TMS Cool Down YouTube Playlist:

https://www.youtube.com/playlist?list=PLYIhIvKYrLX7Fzwk6T_zOV6kI0FYfssti

TMS Legs YouTube Playlist:

https://www.youtube.com/playlist?list=PLYIhIvKYrLX7aXbLeqlT_rJB85P3rFYb9

TMS Upper Body YouTube Playlist:

https://www.youtube.com/playlist?list=PLYIhIvKYrLX7k8qwekQ0k8vO2uxLQA0oL

TMS Core YouTube Playlist:

https://www.youtube.com/playlist?list=PLYIhIvKYrLX4E7YDwht8GHhxTjj5NKeke

TMS Cardio YouTube Playlist:

https://www.youtube.com/playlist?list=PLYIhIvKYrLX4I8zcEBDwdq-eUz0ZdPPxk

TMS Resistance Bands Full Body YouTube Playlist:

https://www.youtube.com/playlist?list=PLYIhIvKYrLX4ChOhYsEA9GvhCBERiYQpj

TMS Fat Loss Training Plan Playlist:

https://www.youtube.com/playlist?list=PLYIhIvKYrLX7IfAQPvp6M4Jz1feUiB_4j

Mix and Match Nutritional Plan Guidelines

https://www.youtube.com/watch?v=PzXmBT-zGTM&t=24s&ab_channel=EmmirMor%C3%A1n

You can also email me at themindsetfitness@gmail.com to receive:

- The list of YouTube playlist exercises ideas

- Fat loss training plan playlist

- Mix and match nutritional meal plan guidelines

- A complimentary copy of *The Mindset 28 Healthy Recipes*. Breakfast, lunch, dinner and snack recipes that are quick and simple.

My Story

Hello, my name is Emmir and I am from Lima Peru. Because I love Frozen Yogurt, I need to active as often as I can, also I love Latin - Afro - Caribbean Music and training in a group and learning from other people.

After overcoming eating disorders and body image confidence, I am a Fat loss Fitness Coach, Speaker, Ex-Fitness model and Founder of The mindset Fitness.

Once upon a time...

Everything started when I moved from Milton Keynes to Bristol, having an *almost clear* idea on how I want to spend my days in this world. Kindly, a commercial gym welcomed me and allowed me to do 6 months of work experience, learning from them and sharing with like-minded people.

After working and studying at the same time for almost 6 months, I received my personal training fitness certificate and for the first time I was able to be part of this amazing team and start helping others.

Nowadays I dedicate my life to the world, sharing my experience and my passion as much as I can. I do not try to preach, propagate or try to convert anyone into fitness. I just know that fitness saved my life when I was on the wrong path and now, I can focus on making a contribution and being a service for anyone who asks for it.

I'm just returning the favour back to life and the universe. Let the universe handle the details and our intentions and desires.

I will release this list of my desires and surrender it to the womb of creation, trusting that when things don't seem to go my way, there is a reason, and that the cosmic plan has designs for me much grander than even those that I have conceived.
The Seven Spiritual Laws of Success by Deepak Chopra.

I'm still learning how to handle those details, it's a process.

My mission is to produce a significant change in the lives of people who ask for my help by enabling the sharing of genuine feelings and providing consideration, positive emotions, honesty, motivation and unconditional love.

Let me contribute, educate and serve you to upgrade your mindset and fitness journey.

To find out more about The Mindset Fitness:
Facebook: https://www.facebook.com/themindsetpt/
Instagram: https://www.instagram.com/themindset_fitness/
Website: www.themindsetfit.com
Email: themindsetfitness@gmail.com

See you soon,
Emmir

Printed in Great Britain
by Amazon